I0413708

Mindfulness for Beginners

How to Live Your Life to the Fullest, Reduce Stress and Find Inner Peace

Jason Andreas

Table of Contents

Introduction

You must have heard this "You need to reduce the stress in your everyday life to live a healthier life", but are you? If you're stressed, anxious, depressed or not at peace; you're going to lower your immune system and open yourself up to a large range of illnesses and ailments, and that is anything from a common cold to heart disease. Lack of concentration and happiness, Anger, weight gain follows along.

You can't be healthy, wealthy or at peace with an unstable mind. That's were living in the present moment or Mindfulness can change your life. Mindfulness will help you to discover your inner peace that will change the course of your life.

If you are willing to change your life and ready to take action towards living a life you deserve, *Mindfulness for Beginners* will guide you through the steps to practicing mindfulness in your day to day life. You can develop life changing mindfulness habits by practicing few minutes each day.

By reading this book, you will learn more about mindfulness, understand what mindfulness really is, why it's important, how it can help you to gain self-awareness, how you can live a life free of stress and anxiety in proven, step by step way —and so much more!

You were always meant to live a peaceful, healthy and a happy life. Read this book and find out how.

Thank you for giving me the opportunity to contribute to your better life.

Chapter 1

What Mindfulness Really Is & What It Means

Have you ever noticed how all of us go through life in a mechanical and robotic manner? All our daily duties are just performed on auto mode and most of the time we aren't really even consciously aware of what we are doing. Even when we eat our meals, we are both sitting and staring at the television or computer as we stuff our faces with much more food than our body actually requires.

We will be physically performing our daily duties and functions but mentally we are somewhere else. While brushing our teeth we will be stressing about the meeting we have later in the afternoon, while driving our kids to school, we are stressing about how we are going to pay for their summer camp and so on.

This happens because we lack the quality of mindfulness. Mindfulness is the state of being conscious or aware of something. It is about being present in the current moment and not dreaming about the future or reminiscing about the past. It is about being aware of exactly what you're doing spiritually, mentally, physically and emotionally.

As the famous Lao Tzu once said, "If you're depressed you're living in the past. If you're anxious you're living in the future. If you're at peace you're living in the present." If you too wish to live a peaceful and content life, it is essential that you live in the present moment. Today we will discuss mindfulness and its meditative techniques and how they can be extremely beneficial to your overall well being and help you turn your life around.

Mindfulness is actually a mindset that allows you to be constantly mindful of what you are doing, but when people commonly refer to mindfulness they are usually referring to meditation techniques that help you to live in the moment. Mindfulness meditation is a combination of techniques that helps to improve your overall physical, spiritual, emotional and mental health. It helps you to understand yourself and keep you grounded and it also plays a major role in eliminating negative energy from your life.

Why is Mindfulness important?

A large number of people go through life in a robotic manner. They mechanically go about performing certain functions and tasks but are absolutely unaware of what they are doing and why they are doing it. In order to live in the present moment, it is absolutely essential for you to be aware of your lifestyle and your actions. You cannot go through life like a robot. Most people focus all their energies on the past or on the future. They forget the beauty and the gift of the present moment. If you truly wish to enjoy the life you need to live in the now. You need to make the most of every moment and you need to indulge in the happiness of the small things. Constantly being mindful can help you become an overall happier and more content human being.

Benefits of Mindfulness

Mindfulness has a large number of benefits and regular and repeated practice of the techniques of mindfulness can be extremely beneficial to your overall being. This book will teach you the various techniques of mindfulness. One of the main benefits is that it can help you reach a more stable state of being. If you are more stable, you're more likely to be calm. Staying calm is going to help you to process everything that is going on around you in the physical world as well as what is going on in your own head.

This will lead to gaining self-knowledge, boosting your immune system, reaching emotional stability and lots of other benefits. From sleeping to starting your day, there is a technique that can help you. From mindfulness of emotions to mindfulness of physical sensation, these techniques only take a few minutes, and the benefits are completely worth the time you invest in the mindfulness techniques.

Best mindfulness technique

The first and most important technique of mindfulness is breathing. Mastering the technique of mindfulness of breathing is an excellent way to keep yourself balanced. The breathing technique helps you keep your mind focused and plays a vital role in eliminating the constant traffic and hustle bustle of your thoughts. The breathing technique plays the most vital role also because it is the one technique that feeds all the other meditation techniques. Here's what you need to know about the breathing technique.

To practice mindfulness of breathing, you need to start by sitting down somewhere where you won't be distracted.

- Next, make sure that you are comfortable and close your eyes. It is usually best if the room is dark. Your breathing is going to be your object of concentration, so start by breathing in through your nose slowly.

- With mindfulness of breathing you won't be following the path of your breath all the way to your lungs, but instead, you are going to make sure that you concentrate on what it feels to take a breath in through your nose.

- Concentrate on how it feels in your nostrils, how it feels for your chest to expand without following the breath. Then, take note of how it feels for that breath to leave your body through your mouth.

- You're going to want to focus on your breathing alone, and some people can do this by counting if they're having trouble.

- It is usually recommended that you count your breathing on each exhale, and count all the way up to ten and then back down again until you get to one.

- This will note the end of your mindfulness of breathing exercise, and you will be able to open up your eyes.

- Some people keep their eyes closed for a moment longer, relishing in the calming and relaxing feeling the body feels.

What does this have to do with your state of being?

The technique of mindfulness of breathing helps you release stress and prevents anxiety. Such release of stress is extremely beneficial to the mind as well as the body. Stress has an extremely negative impact on the spiritual, emotional, physical and mental well-being. All of these aspects of your mind and body need to be in excellent condition in order for you to perform your best and achieve all your goals and desires.

- **Note:** All you need to do is religiously and regularly practice these techniques of mindfulness to achieve success. You can practice one technique a day or maybe even more than one. Some people even practice a single technique more than once a day in order to lock in multiple benefits from the technique. These techniques also help with psychological issues such as anger, anxiety, phobias and other ailments.

Does mindfulness come naturally?

For some people, these techniques come as naturally as breathing after their first session. However, you will find that for the majority of people the act of being mindful and using these techniques is something that is accomplished through discipline, practice and time. It is not something that will come immediately and naturally to you, but practice and discipline will make it easy. It'll be hard to stay focused at first, and this is why it is important to learn tips and tricks along the way. Master mindfulness of breathing before you move forward, as it'll help you to move onto other techniques which may be harder or require more concentration.

Does mindfulness improve your life immediately?

Most people are under the impression that practicing these techniques will have an instant and dramatic effect on their lives. On the contrary, it is only regular and long term practice of these techniques that will bring about gradual and permanent positive changes in your life. Regular practice of these techniques will shift your mindset to a more positive one and help you grow into a better, more successful and content human being. The pace at which this technique changes your life is purely dependent on how often you practice the technique and what your purpose behind using the technique is.

The number of minutes or hours a day you spend practicing these techniques is directly proportionate to your results. The more time you spend practicing these techniques, the faster you will notice the results. Practicing more than just one of these techniques will have a much more profound impact in your life. You will find that various areas of your life are transitioning in a smooth and happy manner.

Chapter 2

Gain Self-Awareness & Understanding

Most people do not really know themselves, who they are, or what really makes them tick. Self-awareness and understand helps you discover your true self. Self-awareness is extremely beneficial because it helps you understand yourself better. It helps you grow in all aspects of your life and you are able to understand your actions and reactions easily. Even those actions and reactions that are absolutely involuntary are far more decipherable to you. You also need to keep in mind that self-awareness is not a static process; it doesn't happen all at once. The longer you spend on these meditative techniques, the more you get to know yourself and things about yourself. There is always something new to learn about yourself.

Importance of self-knowledge

Self-knowledge is something that most people don't have, but there are many benefits to gaining it, such as being able to understand your own emotions. Many people just feel emotions without understanding them, and being aware of emotions can really help you. However, mindfulness of emotions is actually meant to help you understand how to accept and move past your emotions.

If you understand yourself, you are much less likely to be frustrated in certain situations and this will help you to process things quicker, easier, and in a far healthier manner. You're much less likely to rely on vices like alcohol, denial, or even drugs. Instead, you'll be able to move past things in a healthy manner as they come up and your coping mechanisms will improve drastically as well.

You'll also be able to understand why certain patterns in your life recur, bringing you clarity on your life. You need clarity to understand how to break out of the awful rut you may be in, but more importantly you need clarity of yourself, which these techniques can provide when practiced properly.

What is the best practice for gaining self-knowledge?

Almost any one of these techniques, when practiced, will help you to gain self-knowledge, but mindfulness of thought is practiced most commonly for this benefit. If you're looking to start a mindfulness of thought session, you should know that it may take a little longer than other techniques. This is because you have to account for the time it takes to observe a million thoughts that cross your mind.

A mindfulness of thought session may last twenty minutes or more. Some people do have sessions that are ten minutes long, but at least fifteen minutes is usually advised.

Just like any of these other exercises, you are going to want to start in a comfortable position with little to no distractions, so that you can peacefully introspect. Start with mindfulness of breathing and when you feel that you have blocked out the external world, you can move onto focusing on your consciousness instead of on the physical sensation of breathing.

Observe what's bothering you or what you're thinking of. You may just be thinking that it's peaceful, and that's fine as well. Do not interact with and ponder on the thought as this can be detrimental to the process. You do not want to change the way you think or you won't be able to observe yourself properly. Allow your thoughts to wander, and there is no reason to try to control them or redirect them.

No matter what comes up try to keep the flow of your thoughts. Do not get exasperated with your thoughts and do not be judgemental of your thoughts. This practice is not meant to be a conversation with yourself. It doesn't matter if your thoughts are cruel or even sad. You need to just let them flow freely. You can later reflect on what you've learned about yourself but do not do that while you are just trying to observe.

Once you begin to feel that your mind is trying to redirect your thoughts in a particular direction, it's time for you to quit your meditation technique. The best way to end your mindfulness of thoughts session is to come back to the breathing technique. While some people choose to sit in silence for a few moments, others prefer to quickly jot down the things that they wish to reflect on later. Writing down the things you wish to reflect on is highly recommended to further understand your thoughts, yourself and your emotions.

How does this help you gain self-knowledge?

What you've learned from yourself will help you to handle everything that is thrown your way. You're going to want to make sure that you reflect on everything if you want to gain the self-knowledge you seek. You may not truly understand how your own brain works, but by observing your thoughts you see patterns in your thinking, and it can help you see cause and effect of what's happening in your life and in your mental and emotional state. Once you recognize these patterns you'll be able to change them or at least accept them, which can help you to change your coping mechanisms as well. This can help you to improve your overall life.

Is there a best time of day to practice mindfulness of thought?

No there is no particular time of day that you have to practice mindfulness of thoughts to reap the benefits that it has to offer. However, many people find that it's easier to practice mindfulness of thought right before bed or right after they get up in the morning. If you choose to practice mindfulness of thought in the morning before you start your day, you're more likely to feel centered and grounded during the day. This will also have a positive impact on your life and how you interact with the world around you, including the people in it.

Chapter 3

Emotional Stability through Mindfulness

Your emotional stability will actually feed into a lot of different aspects of your life no matter if it's spiritual, physical, or mental. It's important that you have emotional stability, but it's actually hard for many people to reach a level of emotional stability that allows them to handle almost any situation in a healthy manner. Mindfulness can help you to reach emotional stability as well, and it's an easy benefit to reach.

Reach emotional stability

By recognizing your emotions without trying to deny them, you are more easily able to accept your emotions. Every emotion should be accepted, no matter if it's justifiable or not. You cannot stop feeling certain emotions if you want to be emotionally stable, but instead, you need to make sure that you can just filter out your negative emotions, accept them, and change your perspective to something a little more positive.

Benefits of a stable emotional state

There are many benefits to stabilizing your emotions, and one of the biggest benefits is that you won't have to deal with negativity hanging over you.

When you have a stable emotional state, you're much more likely to view the world in a positive manner. You'll be able to filter out negative emotions, and you'll be able to handle difficult situations with a little more ease.

It'll even help you in times of anger, and it'll help you to forgive people. You may not want to forgive people, but keep in mind that when you have a forgiving nature you will have reduced levels of stress. This is because when you're holding a grudge you're spending time and energy on people who don't deserve it, but when you're free from judgment and grudges your mind and soul are at peace.

Is there a mindfulness meditation that is best for your emotional state?

Yes, there actually is. You'll want to practice mindfulness of emotions if you want to get the best results when centering yourself and stabilizing your emotional state. Emotional stability has many benefits, but it can be hard to achieve without proper guidance. Mindfulness of emotion is a great way for you to guide yourself through your emotions and learning to work on them one at a time.

From acceptance to changing your perspective on your emotions, mindfulness of emotions can help you with it all. Over time when you practice it regularly, the practice becomes a part of your identity. This is the increased stability of your emotional state, and it means that it'll be both easier to manage and upkeep.

7 Steps To emotional mindfulness

1. Like all of these meditation forms, you need to start by relaxing and getting comfortable. Make sure that there is no tension in your shoulders, so make sure to be in a comfortable position and then close your eyes.

2. You'll need to focus internally, so don't let the external world distract you. Try to be in a quiet environment, and start with basic breathing exercises. Count your breaths one to ten. Make sure to breathe in through your nose and out through your mouth, paying attention to how it feels for that breath to go from your nostrils to your lungs and back out again.

3. Once your attention is finally focused you can then turn your attention to any strong emotion that you're feeling at the time. This can be anything from anger to anxiety to happiness. You can use both positive and negative emotions. Pick an emotion you're either feeling or a strong one you can pull up. Pull up the memory of what caused that emotion so that you can truly connect with it.

4. Keep your eyes closed and your focus on that emotion, trying to recall everything that led up to it, including any senses you may remember. Imagine the situation, walking yourself through it all over again.

5. You'll feel a tingly sensation in your body. Allow thoughts to enter your mind. Do not entertain the thoughts, and just let them pass by. Ask yourself what emotion you're feeling and if there is more than one.

6. Try to look at the event in a curious manner, looking to see what caused everything to happen. This will prevent you from denying the emotion.

Recognize any physical sensation that is happening as well, such as if your heart is pounding or your muscles are tensing up. This will help you to become more aware, but never judge the emotion. Remember that you shouldn't feel guilty or stressed over this emotion and tell yourself that it's natural.

7. When you feel you have accepted the emotion you should go back to concentrating on your breathing. Then you can open your eyes.

Will you see effects from practicing mindfulness of emotion right away?

Although this technique will bring about a certain amount of emotional stability instantly, it will be a long time before you reach complete emotional stability. You need to repeatedly practice the meditative techniques on a regular basis in order to achieve best results. Repeated and regular practice of this technique will eliminate negativity from your life, thus preventing depression, anxiety, stress and other psychological issues.

When is the best time to practice this type of meditation to help?

You can practice mindfulness of emotion anytime if you want to cultivate a stable emotional state. Of course, you'll also want to make sure you practice it on a regular basis, and doing so at least once a day is recommended. If you feel a particularly strong emotion then you can choose to accept that emotion and learn from it so long as you accept the emotion. Mindfulness of emotion is meant to help you accept these emotions and balance your overall emotional state.

Chapter 4

Strengthen Personal Relationships

One of the biggest issues in any relationship is the conflicts that you're bound to get into. Of course, there can be multiple reasons that your personal relationships are suffering and there are many different types of personal relationships. You have to be in a good place mentally, emotionally and physically if you want to hold yourself in any personal relationship. Practicing these meditative techniques will help you find balance and gain a more positive outlook towards life.

Mindfulness in personal relationships

You'll find that this practice will help you with any of your personal relationships for a wide range of reasons, but one of the main reasons is that it will help you is because it helps you to understand yourself a little better. The more time you spend with these meditation practices, the more you'll be able to learn about yourself. This is how you gain self-knowledge. When you understand a little more about yourself, such as faults, strengths and even issues that you may not yet have resolved, you'll be able to stop taking out your frustrations on other people.

In order to maintain a healthy relationship, it is essential that you handle the problems in the relationship with utmost care. You need to be able to maturely communicate with the opposite person in a manner that's effective and understanding. Now in order to be able to do this, it is necessary for you to first identify the problem. Identification of the problem becomes makes it much easier to resolve any relationship and personal issues. Understanding and regularly practicing these techniques will also help you to let go of all the grudges that you have weighing you down emotionally. You will be able to see the bigger picture and resolve the problem with more clarity and calmness.

If you're going to remain wrapped up and consumed by the thoughts of the event you will not be able to see the bigger picture clearly. There is a possibility that you may be partly or completely at fault but are unable to recognize it due to your clouded vision. In order for you to achieve clarity on the situation, you need to recognize your thoughts and emotions without getting misguided by them or lost in them.

Your thoughts, feelings, and emotions will always have a role to play, but pondering on them will only be adding fuel to the fire. That fire will eventually get so out of control that putting it out will become nearly impossible. It may even end up damaging you on a spiritual and emotional level, which in turn can damage your physical health too. You need to emotionally and mentally clear when analyzing a problem in a relationship otherwise you will only end up blaming the opposite person. The calmer and more collected you are when taking care of a relationship problem, the greater the chances of being able to resolve the issue.

Will this practice help you to forgive the people in your life?

Yes, the regular and repeated practice of these meditative techniques will help you forgive and will also help you let go of things. These techniques help you understand why certain issues crop up and also allow you to handle the situation in a more mature and spiritually evolved fashion. You will be able to clearly see your faults and work on improving them rather than just passing the buck on to the other person in the relationship.

This technique plays a vital role if you're looking to forgive someone. The question of forgiveness only arises when there is negativity and a large number of negative emotions. Anger, jealousy, frustration and other such emotions can create a situation where forgiveness may be required. Whatever negative emotion you're feeling, ensure that you draw it up when practicing the technique of mindfulness of emotions. Focus on the person you need to forgive in order to resolve any issues in the relationship.

Let everything but that person and the anger you feel towards them fade from your mind. Your thoughts will still play out the situation, but observe them without interacting. Pay attention to the emotions you feel when you're face to face with that person, but don't act upon those emotions. Observe the emotions looking at that person's face causes you, but don't fuel those emotions or interact with them.

Tell yourself that you forgive that person. Tell them that they can no longer hurt you. That you'll let the anger go. You may have to repeat it a few times if you want to truly let it take effect. Now, concentrate on your breathing as you turn that mantra inward. Make sure that you concentrate on any residual anger that you are feeling towards them while you're breathing in and out.

With each breath imagine that anger leaving your body and continue to keep your eyes closed. Concentrate on how the breath travels from your nostrils to your lungs, expanding your chest and leaving your lungs. As you exhale, remove the anger along with the breath. Keep this up until you truly feels like you forgive the person, and then you can open your eyes.

How else does mindfulness help with personal relationships?

Mindfulness of emotions helps to keep you stable, grounded and balanced. It will help you have a more positive outlook towards life and towards your emotions. Repeated and regular practice of these techniques will help you stay spiritually, emotionally, mentally and physically well balanced.

This practice has proven to boost the immune system, relieve stress and anxiety and also eliminate all kinds of negative thoughts and emotions. The more positive you are, the better you will react to the situations and circumstances around you. Positivity will also attract more positivity in your life. The positivity you feel and express will spread to all the areas of your life, helping you grow and become the best version of yourself.

How do you reap this benefit from practicing mindfulness?

Now keep in mind that the benefits of practicing mindfulness will only materialize when you follow the practice regularly. If you're expecting an instant reaction and dramatic change in your life it's not going to happen. If you are under the impression that your love life will see an immediate improvement and your problems with loved ones will just vanish, you're wrong. If you want the problems and hassles in your relationship to vanish you need to religiously practice these meditative techniques. You will gradually feel more positive and calm. Patience plays a very important role in mindfulness.

Chapter 5

Help Yourself in Moments of Anger

Anger is something that affects everyone from time to time, and you need to know how to handle it properly if you want to live a healthy life. Anger affects our overall mood, and it can lead to unnecessary stress and anxiety. Of course, these techniques can help with your moments of anger as well. It can help you to walk away from a frustrating and anger-producing situation, but it can also help you reach a type of stability in your inner self that will prevent you from getting angry in the first place.

Isn't anger natural?

Yes, anger is natural and it does need to be accepted. However, there is a difference between accepting your anger and acting on your anger. When you are at the moment, you're more likely to act on your anger than accept it. Anger has many negative effects on your life and you should make sure that you try and balance out these negative effects.

Anger can affect your family as well, as it makes you feel worse, which makes you more likely to lash out at others. If you are feeling down or negative, that will affect those around you as well. You need to feel more positive if you want positivity in your life. Anger can even affect your health, such as your heart health. It can raise your risk of stroke, heart attack, and high blood pressure. It's best to stay away from anger whenever possible, and you should never dwell on anger. It can help with both limiting your anger as well as accepting it so that you can move forward with your life.

How does this technique help you in moments of anger?

This can be a tricky question because it's hard to handle anger when you're in the moment. However, it does a good job at guiding you along the way. The act of being mindful is to be aware of your mental, physical, emotional and spiritual state. Your entire being will go out of balance when you're angry, and these techniques, including meditation, are meant to help put you back into balance.

This is not any different when dealing with anger, but the process is a little harder to handle. Practicing this technique before you try to use it to help your anger is best because it will help you to understand the process and go into the needed state of mind even when you're angry or when you're in a state of emotional distress.

7 Step Mindfulness methods to control Anger

1. You'll want to make yourself aware of the anger that you're feeling and you need to turn inward to see what physical sensation is going through you. Make your mind aware of what your body is going through because during anger it is too likely that you'll separate your body and mind to help you cope with the rage that you're feeling.

2. You may notice sensations in your face, chest, or even your stomach. Your heart rate or breathing may increase and your muscles are likely to tense up. Make sure to observe any and all reactions in your body.

3. Next, you need to remind yourself to breathe, just like you would during mindfulness of breathing. Breathe in and imagine that breath going to where you're feeling these physical sensations, cleansing the area. You can close your eyes if it makes it easier and for many people, it will.

4. Start to count each breath you take, and keep counting until you get to ten. Imagine that every time you breathe out a little more of that anger is released from your body.

5. Keep up with the sensation of breathing as well as the sensations that you are feeling from anger. Observe these sensations as they increase or lessen, and learn to accept it.

6. Next, you'll start to turn more inward, allowing yourself to actually notice your thoughts. You may think your situation isn't fair and that you have a right to be mad, and that you can't take anymore. Any and all thoughts you have don't need to be justified. You just need to accept these thoughts. Let them pass through your mind, but try not interact with these thoughts or you'll end up dwelling on them and increase your anger and frustration.

7. This will help you to dissipate most of your anger. Once you feel your anger under control, you'll be able to see exactly what you're doing in the situation, even if it's not yet clear what you should do next. With most of the anger out of your system, you can then look for a solution and communicate a little better. Remember to stay honest and cope with your anger whenever it occurs.

Does this need to be done on a regular basis?

You can practice any of these techniques on a regular basis, but that doesn't mean you have to practice the technique every single day. It will help if you practice mindfulness of emotion every day because it will help you to learn and accept your emotions, including anger in an easier way. This will help you to control anger as it rises up in the moment as well as deal with the after effects of anger much easier.

The above-mentioned technique can be used each time you find yourself angry. Using this method will help you control your anger better and resolve the issue at hand faster. You will be able to understand why you are angry and how to solve the problem at hand. It is necessary to know what's triggering off the anger in order to solve the problem. Not getting to the root of the cause will only worsen your anger and make it more difficult for you to control your mind in the situation.

Chapter 6

Double Your Concentration

It can also help to boost your overall concentration, and this can help you in many facets of your life. Concentration will help you to succeed in many different ways, including business and school. If you have increased concentration, you are more likely to accomplish anything you put your mind too. This is because you'll be able to put more of your mind into everything you're doing and you're much less likely to become distracted by simple things.

You don't need to have ADD or ADHD to become distracted, but even if you do, these meditative techniques can actually help with such psychological disorders too. It's just a little harder, and it might take a little longer to see some results if you suffer from an actual disorder. Everyone can use a concentration boost, and with these practices that boost can come easy.

Increased concentration for success

When your focus and concentration is increased, as stated above, you're much more likely to succeed in anything that you try to do. When you're trying to learn a new hobby, for example, you'll find that it takes concentration to gain the knowledge needed. It also takes concentration to practice many hobbies, such as wood working, leather working, jewelry making, writing or even embroidery. It doesn't matter what your hobby is, but if you can focus on it attentively, you will get better at your hobby.

You'll also find that you'll be able to reach personal goals that you set if you can concentrate on these meditative practices on a daily basis. This is because procrastination is reduced with the help of these techniques, assisting you to accomplish more, which will, in turn, give you a feeling of accomplishment and happiness.

For example, if you're reading, you'll find that concentration will help you to read a little faster. If you're typing, you'll find that if you focus on what you're typing, you're probably going to type faster. This will help you get your work done faster, and it'll help you to gain knowledge for work or just about anything faster.

You'll still have the ability to multi-task and concentration will actually help with that as well. If you can concentrate on one particular activity, you're more likely to be able to concentrate on a variety of activities because your mind is trained towards focusing.

What mindfulness method is best when you're trying to increase concentration?

There isn't any particular method that will help you with concentration more than others. Instead, you'll find that just about any one of these techniques will help you to concentrate naturally. You'll learn how to block out the external world, and this means that you'll even be able to block out all distractions and focus only on what you're working on. This is demonstrated when you're using mindfulness of breathing and that's because you're concentrating on the physical sensation of breathing.

Concentrating on physical sensation is one way to immerse yourself in anything that you're doing. Take typing for example; if you can immerse your mind in the feeling of typing, then you're more likely to keep typing without distraction. You'll be able to observe the thoughts that come to mind as you write, but you won't have to interact with them. Instead, you'll just transcribe the thoughts that are relevant by typing them, helping you to succeed in what you were trying to type up.

Are there any other ways that mindfulness will help you to concentrate better?

Yes, it will help you to concentrate by removing stress and anxiety naturally. When you're mentally or emotionally unstable, then you won't be able to concentrate on anything that you're doing physically. Your mind won't even be able to hold a thought most of the time, no less acting on something that will lead to success.

Instead, you need to calm your mental and emotional state so that you can reach a stable point which will allow you to work. Just choose a technique, whichever one you feel is most applicable and use it to calm your mental state and balance out your energies.

If you really feel too unbalanced, going and practicing any one of these meditation methods in nature can help. Nature is naturally calming, and it can act as a stress buster. Remember that stress can actually block concentration, just like anxiety and depression. This is why you should never let your emotional state build up until it's out of control. Handle everything as it comes, and you'll find that your mindfulness sessions can be shorter even though they're a little more frequent.

This makes them that much more effective, helping you to reap the benefits of everything that this practice has to offer. You can concentrate on mindfulness of breathing if you want to clear your thoughts, or you can use mindfulness of emotion if something specific is bothering you, but mindfulness of physical sensation can help as well which is where you take stock of everything that is affecting your body, including the tension and aches that you feel.

Does it help if you practice this technique regularly?

Just like if you're practicing mindfulness regularly for any other benefit that it has to offer, you'll find that practicing it regularly will also help you with concentration. It'll become easier and easier to concentrate the more you practice, as your mind is a muscle that you can exercise. Concentration is one of those things that take practice, and your focus can actually sharpen over time. This is why it can help you find a permanent solution to concentration and focus problems, even if you're suffering from a medical condition like ADD or ADHD. Just remember that it may take weeks to notice a difference, but some people will notice a difference in days.

Chapter 7

Strengthen Your Immune System

Now that you know what this meditation technique really is, you're probably wondering how mindfulness can help you. It can actually help your physical health and this is because mindfulness can truly help your immune system. If you have a bad immune system it's important that you add mindfulness to your daily regime. Of course, it's helpful even if you have a decent immune system.

How to improve the immune system?

In time you'll learn these techniques are a form of meditation that will help you to reduce your stress and improve your immune system. It doesn't matter what particular technique you're going to use. What matters is that you use one and doing so on a regular basis is what will help you to reap the benefit of this form of meditation.

Is there another reason that mindfulness helps your immune system?

Yes, there is another reason that this practice is believed to help your immune system, and that's because as you turn your mind inward you become more in tune with your body mentally and physically. This allows your mind to be more aware of any illness you may be feeling, even on a subconscious level.

Many people believe that this is one of the reasons that the immune system may improve, help us to fight off any illness as it comes. You're more likely to notice small symptoms of illness when you are practicing mindful meditation because you'll notice your body as a whole. You'll be able to tell if your throat is slightly sore, if your muscle aches if you're feeling hotter than usual and so on.

Your mental state is also known to affect your immune system. If you are more positive, your immune system is higher because there is less holding it down. If you are experiencing emotional trauma, even subconsciously, you will hamper your immune system because the effects of anxiety will sink in, which can also lead to depression.

Mindfulness meditation, just like meditation as a whole, is known to help produce more antibodies and stimulate the immune system regions of the brain. This helps to stimulate your immune system as a whole. However, the effects aren't immediate, and sometimes a noticeable effect will take up to eight weeks.

What are the benefits of a raised immune system?

If you have a healthy immune system, you will have reduced stress levels. This means that you're more likely to be a more positive person. You're also more likely to be able to handle the disappointments that come to you without falling into depression or experiencing too much anxiety about small issues. With a healthy immune system, one of the most obvious and noteworthy benefits is that you won't be prone to getting sick.

This is useful all year round, but you'll also find that it's extremely useful during flu and cold season. If you get sick, you're more likely to fall into a rut, feel depression, miss work, lack concentration, and feel generally frazzled, making your quality of life go down. It can be hard to recover from being sick both physically and mentally, but with this form of meditation creating a boosted immune system, you're much more likely to be able to avoid the entire ordeal.

Does it matter what mindfulness meditation that you use?

No, it doesn't matter what type of meditation technique you use. All forms of meditation are meant to center you and this is what will help you boost your immune system. Of course mindfulness of breathing is one of the easiest exercises to work into your daily routine. Just make sure that you have at least ten minutes dedicated to these exercises.

There are different varieties of these practices that can be implemented to reach the benefit of a raised immune system, and it doesn't even matter where you practice. You can practice on the bus, at home, and even in nature. Adding nature into your mindfulness meditation practice will help as well since nature is also known to help boost the immune system as well as improving your general attitude.

Does it have to be done in a routine to achieve this benefit?

Yes, to achieve this benefit you do need to make a routine of it. It is best to practice one of these techniques at least once daily for any benefit that it has to offer. However, you'll find that if you're trying to boost your immune system all you need to do is practice at least once daily for ten to fifteen minutes. You can improve your chances of boosting your immune system drastically by practicing in nature, in a quiet place, or more than once daily. Just remember that the effects of a boosted immune system do not show immediately, and just because you are unsure if it is working doesn't mean you should stop your practices. Instead, keep it up, as it may take up to eight weeks to notice an effect.

Chapter 8

Reach Your Weight Loss Goals

Everyone has a few weight loss goals every once in a while. Some people want to lose more weight than others and that's fine. No matter how much or how little weight you want to lose, you'll want to use these meditative techniques to help reach your weight loss goals. There are many different techniques that you can use to help you reach every weight loss goal you have.

Lose weight being mindful

It is known to reduce stress, which will help you to lose weight. When you are less stressed, you're less likely to be anxious or depressed. Anxiety or depression can also lead to weight gain and these techniques can help in getting rid of your anxiety, thereby having a positive impact on your weight. You need to center yourself, and then you'll be able to help improve your overall mood and energy levels. When you're more positive, you have more energy in the first place.

How much weight can you lose?

It can help you reach all of your weight loss goals and it's great in helping you to maintain the weight you want as well. Basic techniques can help you maintain your weight because it reduces your stress. Stress has been proven to worsen weight gain as well as self-control, which will lead to mindless eating that will also make you put weight on. There will be a point that weight loss will lessen and seem to come to a plateau when you're using any of these techniques to help you lose weight, but if you're patient you'll be able to push past it to lose more weight so long as you're practicing it with a healthy lifestyle as well.

What mindfulness practice is best to help you lose weight?

Mindfulness of eating practices are the best to help you lose weight. Many people aren't aware of just how much they're eating and many people will sit down and eat a bag of chips without realizing exactly what they've done and how many calories they've consumed. This is one of the main reasons that people tend to gain weight. Mindfulness of eating will help you to enjoy your food while you are still making sure that everything you eat is controlled, even the junk food.

Mindfulness of eating is the act of eating with your five senses.

7 Steps to mindful eating

1. Take a small bite of food and take it with you, sitting down comfortably.

2. Next, you're going to want to turn off any distractions. Make sure that you tune out the external world, and mindfulness of breathing is usually the best way to center yourself so that you're not distracted.

3. Then start by smelling your food. Enjoy the scent of what the food smells like. Concentrate on what the food feels like in your fingers or when placed to your lips. Look at the food, and take note of how appetizing the food looks to you.

4. If there's any sound, try to appreciate that sound like if a bag is crinkling, and then once you've appreciated the food, take a small bite of it.

5. No matter how small the food piece is, try to make it at least two bites. Savor the food, chewing slowly. Eat only a few bites at a time and you will feel far more satisfied than if you were eating mindlessly.

6. Concentrate on how the taste lingers on your tongue as you transitioning yourself back to breathing and then open your eyes to go back about your day.

7. It may sound quite funny while you read but if you practice mindfulness of eating, you're much less likely to mindlessly eat and gain weight.

So do you need to use a proper diet and exercise, or is mindfulness enough?

It is a great way to get a head start on your weight loss goals, but it's not enough to help you lose all of the weight you want. You may lose a few pounds with this technique on its own, but you'll never lose a lot without a proper diet and exercise. Remember that exercise will help to boost your metabolism, making all of your weight loss efforts that much more effective. Burn off the calories you eat, even when you are using mindfulness of eating practices. A proper diet is also necessary because you won't lose weight if you're eating foods that are bad for you and even if you do lose weight by cutting back on the amount you consume, it won't be sustainable weight loss on its own.

Weight loss results

Will you see results quickly or does it take a while when trying to lose weight with mindfulness?

Sadly, actual weight loss will take time, just like any other method of weight loss. However, you should notice that you feel much more satisfied after you use mindfulness of eating and you're more likely to appreciate your food more as well. This will mean that you won't have to eat as much to feel as satisfied. You will even find yourself satisfied with smaller amounts of food than usual and you will end up eating smaller quantities of food than you originally did. You will stop eating out of boredom and eat only to keep your stomach filled and your overall health excellent.

If you eat too quickly, it's proven that you're more likely to eat too much. You can practice mindfulness of eating anytime you want to, and some people even practice a session during every meal. Just make sure that you aren't eating with distraction because it will pull you out of your exercise and negate the positive effects that you'd get from it.

This is why eating in a room by yourself or at least at a table without any distractions, such as TV or the computer, is usually recommended when you're trying to lose weight. It doesn't matter if you exercise before mindfulness of eating, but many people still prefer exercising afterward so they can burn off the calories. The positivity will also tend to give you more energy for your exercise routine.

Chapter 9

Help Your Sleep & Dreams

Everyone knows that sleep is extremely important and dreams are important too. You'll feel more positive when you have enough sleep and you've had positive dreams. Luckily, if you are more positive overall, positive dreams will come naturally as well. Experiencing a positive dream cycle will help you to feel more rested at night and the amount of sleep you get will affect every aspect of your life. If you're too tired, you're much more likely to do poorly in work, school or even at social events. Negativity can hang on your energy if you aren't getting enough sleep and lack of sleep can lead to a variety of medical problems as well.

Importance of a peaceful sleep

As stated above, one of the main benefits of getting enough sleep and dreaming during it is that you'll be able to act more positively and view the world in a more positive manner. Better sleep will also help to ease chronic pain, improve the functioning of your heart and overall health. If you're getting enough sleep you're also less likely to become injured because sleep deprivation can cause many disasters, including car accidents.

It'll increase your general mood and positivity, which will help you to be more productive and reach whatever goals that you put out and it'll help you to keep your weight under control. Sleep and good dreams lower your stress, which is also needed for positive interactions. You're also able to make better decisions when you have a good night's sleep because you have a clearer head and you will be less irrational. Not to mention that it can improve your immune system as well as your memory.

How does it help your sleep and your dreams?

You may be wondering how this meditation form will help you to dream better and improve your sleeping pattern. One of the main ways is that it removes anything that is stressing you out to the point that you can't sleep. With these practices, you'll learn how to remove these stress factors and it can even help your aches and pains. For example, one of the main reasons that people have trouble sleeping is that a problem they are facing is stressing them out.

It is also known to help you with clarity, and you'll want to try mindfulness of breathing to help relax you as well. The clarity you gain from these practices will help you to put your problems into perspective.

If you're feeling angry at a particular person, you can also use mindfulness of emotions to help. This version of mindfulness that helps with forgiveness is also best if you're trying to make yourself forgive someone so that they stop affecting your sleep and dreams. If you're having too many nightmares, mindfulness of breathing before bed for anxiety reasons is usually recommended.

7 steps for a peaceful sleep

As stated above, mindfulness of breathing and mindfulness of emotions is going to help you get a good night's sleep. However, you'll find that mindfulness of physical sensation is extremely helpful when you are trying to get to sleep. You'll need at least fifteen minutes to do it, but the process is actually pretty easy.

1. Just start by closing your eyes after you've found a comfortable position to sit in. Focus all of your attention on mindfulness of breathing at first, and experience the breathing. You should feel yourself riding each of your breaths as if you were riding waves, and pay attention to how it moves through your body.

2. Afterward, you'll want to shift your awareness to the feel of sitting. Pay close attention to how it feels to sit in the chair.

3. Notice all of the parts that are in contact with the chair. Try to immerse yourself in that feeling, and allow yourself to just exist in that moment.

4. Next, start to take stock of your body, and allow yourself to expand your awareness to your body as a whole. Recognize if there is a breeze against your arms if you feel cold, or even if there are any aches or pains in your body. Notice if you're experiencing thirst or hunger. Make sure to take stock of all of the physical sensations that you're feeling.

5. Remember that you should never judge any experience, just like you wouldn't judge any emotion. You also don't want to label any sensation because this will snap you out of your physical awareness, and you shouldn't hunt for a sensation. Don't ask yourself if you are hungry, but instead, just take note of it if you notice it when you expand your consciousness.

6. Allow yourself to feel all of that and once you feel you've fully immersed yourself into a physical sensation for a little while, try and shift your attention back to how it feels for your body to make contact with the chair.

7. Then, shift it to how it feels to breathe. Allow yourself to feel that once more for a few moments before you open your eyes.

Is there a best time to practice mindfulness of physical sensation to improve your sleep and dreams?

Yes, the best time to practice mindfulness of physical sensation is right before you go to bed. This will help you to relax and it'll help you to release any tension that you may be having. This should allow you to drift off to sleep without anything bothering your mind, consciously or subconsciously. Of course, other exercises can also be performed throughout the day and right up to bedtime to help you with better sleep and dreams as well.

Chapter 10

Always Keep These Tips & Tricks in Mind

There are still tips and tricks to mindfulness that you can apply if you're having trouble, as it'll help to ease you into the process as well as help you to just understand mindfulness as a whole. Once you've mastered mindfulness of breathing, everything else should come a little more naturally, but that doesn't quite make it natural.

Avoid Jewelry

It may seem strange at first, but it is usually best that you avoid jewelry if you're trying to practice any of these mindful techniques. This is because jewelry is distracting. It is shiny if you have your eyes open, heavy, jingles, and it can sometimes pinch. This is more likely to make you aware and keep you aware of the physical world around you when you are trying to pull your thoughts somewhere else so that you can practice a technique. You can just temporarily remove this jewelry as it's better if the distraction isn't there when you get started.

Avoid Uncomfortable Clothing

Uncomfortable clothing should be avoided for the same reason that you'd want to avoid jewelry when you're trying to practice any of these techniques. This is because any of these practices and techniques require concentration on a specific aspect of what you are feeling, experiencing, or doing. You do not want to be distracted by something that is pinching you, too tight, or making you feel suffocated. Yoga pants are actually recommended, but anything you feel comfortable in will do. Remove things like belts or uncomfortable shoes before starting any exercise or technique.

Practice One Technique at a Time

Don't try to move onto other mindfulness techniques unless you have really mastered mindfulness of breathing. Mindfulness of breathing is like your foundation that will help you build up your knowledge of mindfulness, helping you to practice it properly. You can then move onto another technique, but never try to really learn more than one at a time. Eventually, you should know every technique that you want to, but you'll find out that it does take time.

Try to Avoid Light

Unless a mindfulness technique requires you to see something, it is usually best to practice in a dark room. This is because even when your eyes are closed, you'll see a red tinge to your eyelids as the light tries to filter through. It is easier for you to concentrate internally if you're not being distracted by lighting. Of course, black out curtains are recommended.

You can practice this meditation form in sunlight, especially if you want to practice outside, but it's not recommended if you're a beginner. If you want to practice outside, try to practice in the shade where the lighting that you're seeing from behind your eyes is less likely to change due to cloud coverage or other shadows flickering through the light.

Remember Not to Judge

Part of being mindful is to live in the moment without judging the moment, and that can be very hard to master. It is human nature to judge and label things including ourselves. If you are truly experiencing the present, you are not allowing yourself to spoil the experience with your judgments. This is why you should try not to judge what you're feeling especially if you are practicing mindfulness of thoughts or emotion. Judging can ruin the entire exercise. Leave your reflections for a later time and simply focus only on your meditative practice.

Get Rid of Negativity as It Comes

It is harder to be mindful and positive if you let negativity build within you or around you. This is why part of being mindful successfully is doing so regularly. If you are experiencing negativity in your emotions, feeling down for some unknown reason, having issues sleeping, experiencing nightmares or anything else that is causing negativity, then practice mindfulness so that you can let it go. Letting it go is important, as it helps you to rebalance yourself, which improves your positivity and reduces stress in your overall life.

Don't Become Frustrated

You need to try and not become frustrated, even if you're having a hard time being mindful. This is because this is a meditation practice that is hard for many people, and you can't expect to be a natural at it. Experiencing true mindfulness will require patience and practice, so you have to have the time to dedicate to it. You won't see immediate benefits, at least not drastic ones, but you will experience these benefits if you practice these methods diligently and successfully. However, if you become frustrated you are allowing negativity and stress to enter your being and your life. This will block you from being mindful successfully. So stick to it, and be patient.

Make a Routine

It is important that you try and make a routine out of any one of these practices. This will help you buckle down and practice like you need to in order to achieve success. It is usually best to practice mindfulness at least once a day and if you set a time aside for it in the first place, you're more likely to stick with it. This will allow you to develop the patience that you need to decrease your stress and increase your positivity.

There is no specific time of day to practice mindfulness, but try doing so at least in the morning or at night. These are the two most successful times to practice mindfulness without interruption. Ensure that you're wide awake before you begin your practice in the morning because the relaxing effects of this meditative technique may put you right back to sleep. For those suffering from sleep disorders and nightmares, it is recommended that they practice the meditative techniques before bedtime to get a good night's sleep.

www.ingramcontent.com/pod-product-compliance
Lightning Source LLC
Chambersburg PA
CBHW071138280526
45787CB00003B/1330

* 9 781534 993631 *